Walking Free

A Journey Into Life In All Its Fullness

Dr. Kate Jutsum

Walking Free: A Journey Into Life In All Its Fullness
Copyright © 2013 by Dr. Katherine Jutsum. All rights reserved.

Published by Akas Creative
www.katejutsum.org

No part of this book may be reproduced, stored in a retrieval system or transmitted in any form or by any means - electronic, mechanical, photocopy, recording, or otherwise - without prior written permission of the copyright owner, except by a reviewer who wishes to quote brief passages in connection with a review for inclusion in a magazine, newspaper or broadcast.

Unless otherwise stated, all Scripture quotations are taken from The Holy Bible, New King James Version (Copyright (C) 1979, 1980, 1982 by Thomas Nelson, Inc.).

Requests for information should be addressed to:
Kate Jutsum
kjutsum@gmail.com

ISBN 978-0-9924380-0-5

Pre-release Edition printed August 2013
Final Edition printed January 2014

WALKING FREE

*To all those courageous enough to
confront their fears and journey
where no-one but God can take them*

WALKING FREE

Contents

Introduction 9
Acknowledgments. 11

Day 1: Hearing God's Voice. 13
Day 2: Transforming Our Minds 17
Day 3: A Battle For Agreement 21
Day 4: Fear vs Faith 25
Day 5: What To Do With Lies 29
Day 6: Declarations. 33
Day 7: Rest 37
Review of the Week **39**

Day 8: A New You 41
Day 9: Who I Am 45
Day 10: Sonship (Part I) 49
Day 11: Sonship (Part II). 53
Day 12: The Power of Gratitude 57
Day 13: The Normal Christian Life 61
Day 14: Love. 65
Review of the Week **69**

Day 15: Community 71
Day 16: Looking After You. 75
Day 17: Embracing Process 79
Day 18: Keeping The Enemy Foothold-Free 83
Day 19: When Trouble Comes 87
Day 20: Looking After Your Spirit 91
Day 21: Onward Development. 95

Appendices
Appendix A: 100
Appendix B: Extra truth sheets 102
Appendix C: Declarations 109
Appendix D: Further Reading and Resources 111
References. 115

Introduction

Shortly into my journey in ministry in inner healing and deliverance I saw a vision of an army camp with round white tents and a small fire just about still alight and soldiers lying, in battle dress but asleep, all over the camp. They looked like they'd come back from battle, exhausted, and had just dropped, their weapons lying around on the ground. Gradually the soldiers started to wake up and get a shower and a change of clothes, then they found their weapons again and started skills-training.

As I mused over what I'd seen, God told me that what I was seeing represented the church. The soldiers are us and the inner healing is the shower and the change of clothes, dealing with the past and the grime from battles gone by, the smell of war, fatigue and actual physical injury, and it's an empowering into a new season. A change into fresh, new clothes that fit perfectly and were always available, but never worn.

Of course that shower and change of clothes is just the beginning. The real reason for the change is the building of an army that is alive, alert, highly skilled and working as a team. The real aim has only ever been revival, or actually, preferably, reformation; a move of God that affects every part of our culture and way of life and brings with it a whole new normal.

The last few years here on this side of the world has shown that we can do showers and clothing changes pretty well, but it has been rather more difficult to help people through to take up their place in the move of God that has started. That is the reason for this booklet.

Whilst research has shown that a great many people never lose the freedom they get from their prayer ministry, there are some things that you can do to make it easier for yourself and to continue to grow.

This booklet aims to consolidate and build on your ministry session, or, if you haven't had one, on truths that God gives you in place of lies you had been believing. It's also about how to play the game of life. Even those who are clean and skilled can go astray if they don't know how battle works, so we'll go through some things to set you up well for your future walk with God.

Be aware that what you get out of this will be proportional to what you put in, so I would encourage you to just take these 21 days as an investment into your future.

You were born for a unique purpose and destiny. No-one else can fill the place God put you on the earth to fill and no-one can love Him like you love Him. The world is waiting to see you in all your glory, unveiled as the son or daughter of God that you are. As you go through this twenty-one days, and the rest of your life, I pray that you grow from glory to glory in leaps and bounds, that you become intimately acquainted with our awesome God and Father, and that at every turn of the path that leads you into the fulfillment of His destiny for you, you are surprised and delighted by His love.

Kate Jutsum
11 June, 2013

With my heartfelt thanks and appreciation
to all those that lent their colour to this project,
and enabled it to happen

WALKING FREE

WALKING FREE

Day 1: Hearing God's Voice

*My sheep hear my voice, and I know them,
and they follow me.*
John 10:27

Do you hear God? The answer to this question, for most Christians, would be 'maybe'. They occasionally hear Him as they read His word, or through preaching, or through a prophetic word, but don't really realise that He's speaking all the time, and that a lot of what He says they're hearing, but dismissing as coincidence, or their own thoughts.

If you are doing this post-ministry session, do you realise that you were hearing God consistently through your session? Every impression, every picture, every word on your truth sheet is evidence of you seeing, hearing and perceiving clearly. As Jesus said in John 10, our natural, 'born-with' normal is to hear God's voice, like sheep know the voice of their shepherd, whether that's through prayer ministry or through every day life. Most of us are hearing Him much more than we realise.

Over the next few days we're going to identify some key truths in your life and use those as a springboard to hear God more, both in those areas and in other areas that crop up. I would urge you to spend time just allowing Him to speak to you, and look out for His nudges through your day (and night!) over the coming weeks. Remember, once He's given you a picture you can go back there and ask Him more questions.

God speaks in images in our mind's eye (commonly called visions), dreams, through scripture, 'coincidence' and circumstance, internal impressions, the world around us, knowledge that just seems to have come from nowhere, and random thoughts that are too good to be yours! In fact, He will speak to us in whatever way we are open to hear Him. God's primary language is not English, and He delights to hide where we can find Him!

Looking into Life

Looking back at your walk with God or ministry session, what ways does He often seem to speak to you?

- ☐ *Mind pictures*
- ☐ *Still small voice*
- ☐ *Impressions*
- ☐ *Circumstance*
- ☐ *Dreams*
- ☐ *Music*
- ☐ *Bible reading*
- ☐ *Other people*
- ☐

What one scene from your session (or previous God-encounters) stands out to you the most?

_____
_____
_____

Go back there... Where is God now? What's He doing? Is there anything He wants to tell you? Spend some time enjoying Him and write down what He tells you.

_____
_____
_____
_____

Sanctified Imagination versus Visualisation

Much concern exists over the imagination in the Christian world. We don't have space here for a full discussion of the topic but I will make two brief comments.

Firstly, our mind has a canvas. It's quite like an iPad actually, in that the same screen can be utilised by many different applications. Our imagination uses our mind's canvas, and so does our memory. If you stop now and imagine a pink elephant and then remember what you had for dinner last night, both pictures settle in the same place in your mind. It stands to reason that God would use the same canvas, given that He created it. It's our job to keep that canvas clean.

Secondly, just because the New Age misuses the imagination in visualisation doesn't mean that we should avoid the imagination completely. The enemy cannot create so he perverts what God has made, and you have to have something real for a counterfeit to exist.

We always need to be Holy Spirit-led in our ventures using that canvas, because of its multi-purpose nature. Let's not give in to the fear of being deceived and, in doing so, deceive ourselves.

Day 2: Transforming Our Minds

*Do not conform to the pattern of this world,
but be transformed by the renewing of your mind.
Then you will be able to test and approve what God's will is
—His good, pleasing and perfect will.*
Romans 12:2

Wouldn't it be wonderful if we could be 'zapped' by God and perfected in a second, with no further issues in life, and with no need for any work on our part? God, intentionally limiting Himself to allow relationship with us, partners with us to see things change. One of the ways He does this is to transform us as we choose to renew our minds. But what does this mind renewal business actually look like?

Whenever something becomes normal it sets up a track in our brains. A habit or thought pattern takes a while to get laid down, but once it's established it's very strong. Mind changes therefore have to be deliberate, and often take work on our parts! If you've ever tried to break a habit you'll know what I mean. The Greek here is anakainōsis; it means 'renovation'. It paints a picture of us being born with an empty house that is gradually decorated by parents, siblings, friends and ourselves during early life. When we come to know Jesus, He takes a walk through our house, decides to redecorate and He radically changes the colour scheme. It takes some readjustment on our part, but if we'll help Him, the renovation will always be beautiful.

18

Our childhoods, up to around ten to fifteen years of age, are all about learning. Pathways are constantly being laid down that we continue to utilise for the rest of our lives. This is great! It means that your school arithmetic is still in there somewhere. But it also means that when we learn lies they're in there too, filtering our view on life. When we choose to renew our minds, it's like deliberately deciding to renovate them. It takes a while to reinforce the new truth, but stick at it and over time, it'll actually become easier to access than the lie was.

Looking into Life

Have a think about, or ask God, what lies you are believing about Him, yourself or the people around you.

_____
_____
_____
_____

What truths does He want to replace those lies with? Write them here:

1. _____

2. _____

3. _____

Were there any truths that you were surprised by?

_____
_____
_____
_____

20

Were there any themes to what God told you?

_____
_____
_____
_____
_____

Were there any areas that weren't dealt with that you still want to ask God about? What's He saying about these?

_____
_____
_____
_____
_____
_____

Declarations

I have the mind of Christ.

I am being transformed day by day as I partner with God to renew my mind.

Day 3: A Battle For Agreement

For we do not wrestle against flesh and blood, but against principalities, against powers, against the rulers of the darkness of this age, against spiritual hosts of wickedness in the heavenly places.
Ephesians 6:12

It has been said that the whole of life is a battle for who and what we are going to agree with. From the time sin came into the world, reality was divided. Now we find ourselves in a world where we are fed news from many sources every day. Consider where you've received information from today: books, the newspaper, radio, television, the internet, friends, magazines, Facebook, billboards… the list is endless. Many sources of information seek to make us agree with them in some way so as to get hold of our hard-earned cash. For example, we choose their laundry powder, or continue to buy their newspaper.

The same battle, though, rages over what we'll give our heart and mind to in the spirit realm. Both God and the enemy have information streams running in our direction; both have their own 'truth'. We have the decision who we're going to partner with. And just as whatever we spend money on finds its way into our homes, so whoever we partner with influences the world around us, be it God or the enemy.

22

We know from Ephesians six that our battle is not against flesh and blood, but against principalities and powers in the heavenly realms. God's aim is that we, as His delegated authority and His kids on the earth, demonstrate Him to those very principalities and powers. But if we're agreeing with their view of the world we are hardly in the position to do that. By agreeing with God we instead open up the realm around us to His invasion, and as His reality becomes more and more real on earth (on earth as it is in heaven), the enemy has to shift, bringing outpourings and revivals. You can see, then, how important it is that we're agreeing with the right news channel.

Looking into Life

Write your first truth from your ministry session here:

_____
_____
_____

Can you remember how God gave you this truth? Was it a sense or a picture, did you hear it or feel it?

_____
_____

What lie was it replacing?

_____
_____
_____

How has it been since you received this truth? Has the lie tried to get you again? How did you do standing on the truth?

_____
_____
_____

Spend a few minutes meditating on (asking God about) this truth. What else did He tell you about it?

_____
_____
_____
_____
_____

What would your life look like in a year if you believed this truth?

_____
_____
_____
_____
_____

What can you declare to reinforce this truth in your life?

_____
_____
_____
_____

Day 4: Fear vs Faith

*For God has not given us a spirit of fear, but of power
and of love and of a sound mind.
2 Timothy 1:7*

When God handed earth over to us as people made in His image to run, it was a total handover. So total, in fact, that when we handed the authority God gave us to the enemy, Jesus had to come as a man to get it back. What we say, what we do and what we think and believe has incredible sway on earth.

We all know God's kingdom runs on faith, which at its simplest is agreement with God that what He says is true. What many of us haven't learned is that fear is to the enemy's world what faith is to God's. That is, any area in life where we are in fear, it's because we're believing what the enemy says over and above what God says. We are agreeing with the enemy at the expense of God's truth. And the problem with that? In agreeing with the enemy, as we learned yesterday, we allow the enemy access into our lives to areas that he didn't previously have access to.

So whoever we agree with, we partner with, and we empower them and allow them access to change our surroundings, whether the enemy through fear or God through faith. With God, our agreement brings whatever is good, lovely, admirable and worthy of praise.

As the one who steals, kills, destroys and divides, what the enemy brings can never be good news.

It is vital to walk in agreement with God—which is called faith—and to shut out every attempt of the enemy to deceive us again.

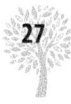

Looking into Life

What main fears have you been set free from during your walk with God or session? Have any of those fears tried to come back since?

_____
_____
_____
_____

What tools did God give you to fight the fear when it comes knocking?

_____
_____
_____
_____

How have you put that advice into practice?

_____
_____
_____
_____

Where is Father God right now? Is there anything else He's telling you about the fear?

_____
_____
_____
_____

What can you do differently when fear comes from now on?

_____
_____
_____
_____

How will your life look different in a year, as you win against the fears that have tried to hold you back?

_____
_____
_____
_____

Day 5: What To Do With Lies

*And you shall know the truth,
and the truth shall make you free.
2 Timothy 3:17*

So you've discovered by now that the enemy loves lies. They have, after all, served him well for a long time. You may have had some of the old lies try to slip in again, or you may even have started to notice other ones that you weren't even aware of before. How have you been responding to them?

Lies can seem so comfortable, so familiar, so like our own thoughts, that it often takes a real effort to see them leave.

So how do we remove them? Well, for a start we have to decide what the truth is, when we are in a calm situation and we trust ourselves to think rationally. I recall a situation in my life where I'd been falsely accused of something quite significant. In my normal, rational state I knew that the accusations were totally wrong, but if I was in a place of stress, sleep deprivation, a negative atmosphere, or hormonal craziness (ladies you know what I'm talking about!), then suddenly every ability of my brain to be rational seemed to totally evaporate. Somehow the enemy's lies seemed to make perfect sense. In that place, if we can look back at something we know was truth when we were of 'sound mind' and just hang on regardless of the buffeting, we'll soon bob back up to the surface of happy lucidity.

Secondly, we need to have a solid grounding in God's word, so that thoughts that sound benign enough can be tested against God's truth. When we find a lie, we can flick it away with truth, or if we know it's wrong but don't know the truth, we can simply laugh at it and ask God what the truth is. By the way, have you tried laughing at lies yet? Steve Backlund, of Bethel Church, has a great book called *Let's Just Laugh At That,* which deals with this very issue. All part of mind renewal.

Looking into Life

Write your second truth from your ministry session here:

_____
_____
_____

Can you remember how God gave you this truth? Was it a sense or a picture, did you hear it or feel it?

_____
_____

What lie was it replacing?

_____
_____
_____

How has it been since you received this truth? Has the lie tried to get you again? How did you do standing on the truth?

_____
_____
_____

Spend a few minutes meditating on (asking God about) this truth. What else did He tell you about it?

_____
_____
_____
_____
_____

What would your life look like in a year if you believed this truth?

_____
_____
_____
_____
_____

What can you declare to reinforce this truth in your life?

_____
_____
_____
_____

Day 6: Declarations

Death and life are in the power of the tongue.
Proverbs 18:21

God, who gives life to the dead and calls those things which do not exist as though they did.
Romans 4:17

Today we're learning another tool on our mind-transformation belt: Declarations!

Making declarations, that is, speaking out loud God's truth over our lives, has many purposes. Firstly, our words have creative power. That means whenever we speak out what God says we're declaring it into existence. Secondly, as we make declarations we're reminding ourselves what truth is. We are reinforcing those brain pathways we mentioned a few days ago.

It is not unusual to hear people say, "But I can't say that I'm walking in signs and wonders, because I'm not. It would be hypocritical."

Is making declarations hypocritical? The story is told of an apple tree. When it is fully grown and covered in apples, it is undeniably an apple tree. How about when it's a sapling? How about the years before it fruits? We'd have to say that it's an apple tree right from day one. We're not about denial here—that helps no-one—but when we make declarations, we're saying, "ok, I know I'm not seeing the fruit of this yet, but God has said that I walk in divine health, so I'm going to partner with Him in agreeing that what He says is true.'"

Some truths are true of every believer, but there are also truths specific to each of us. God, treating each one of us as His favourite, interacts with each of us according to our individual make-up. That means He treats each of us differently, because we're all unique.

You can see some example declarations in Appendix C.

Looking into Life

Write your third truth from your ministry session here:

_____
_____
_____

Can you remember how God gave you this truth? Was it a sense or a picture, did you hear it or feel it?

_____
_____

What lie was it replacing?

_____
_____
_____

How has it been since you received this truth? Has the lie tried to get you again? How did you do standing on the truth?

_____
_____
_____

Spend a few minutes meditating on (asking God about) this truth. What else did He tell you about it?

_____
_____
_____
_____
_____

What would your life look like in a year if you believed this truth?

_____
_____
_____
_____
_____

What can you declare to reinforce this truth in your life?

_____
_____
_____
_____

Day 7: Rest

*He makes me to lie down in green pastures.
He leads me beside the still waters, He restores my soul;
He leads me in the paths of righteousness for His name's sake.
Psalm 23:2-3*

Have you ever done a fitness program? You know the sort where they tell you what exercises to do every day to get you fit in a short amount of time? What one thing do you find in every exercise program? Apart from hundreds of sit-ups and way too much running up hills, that is! It's a rest day.

Science, in my definition being a study of the mind of God, has come to the same conclusion that God set out from the beginning of time: Our bodies need rest. And it will come as no surprise that our minds, souls and spirits need rest as well.

The reason for rest in a fitness program isn't just to be nice so you'll keep up with the program, although psychologically rest certainly helps. It's because when we exercise our muscles get damaged at a micro-level. These tiny muscle tears (which cause the soreness we often feel after a good workout) are fine, but without rest to allow repair significant damage can occur at a whole-muscle level.

Our whole being works just the same. Daily life causes micro-tears in our minds, spirits and souls. Unless someone looks very closely they won't see anything, but give it enough time without rest and those little things become all too obvious to everyone! Whilst that can look like an outburst of anger, it may be as subtle as the gradual in-creeping of hopelessness, the slipping of quality time with God, or a growing irritation towards people and situations.

God has a place of rest for each one of us to go to all through life. It is vital that we learn where that is and how to access it regularly, so that we stay in a place of excellent spiritual and emotional health.

What does rest look like?

Imagine lying back in a hot tub, contemplating the universe as the warm water moves around you. Is that rest to you? For some people, relaxing in a hot tub is the epitome of rest. For doers though, nothing could be more stressful! Rest for them looks like walking or doing photography, or fixing up a car. Anything but sitting still! So what is rest? Well, you won't be surprised to hear that, whilst we all need periods of relaxation away from 'work', whatever that looks like to us, rest is actually an inside job. Less a day in seven, and more a twenty-four-seven state of 'being' in which we are in a place of total trust and security in God and our internal world is at peace as a result.

Review of the Week

What are you thankful for this week?

_____
_____
_____
_____

What aspects of God have you seen in action?

His love for me	His restoration	His grace
His goodness	His provision	His beauty
His faithfulness	His forgiveness	His comfort
His strength	His peace	His power

Spend a few minutes with God, remembering what He's done and who He is and thanking Him for how He's shown Himself to you this week. Write down anything He says to you here:

_____
_____
_____
_____

Are there any people that you need to forgive? Spend some time praying through this.

_____
_____
_____
_____

Are there any situations in the coming week you want to run past Him? Write down what He says here:

_____
_____
_____
_____
_____

Day 8: A New You

*Therefore if anyone be in Christ, he is a new creation.
The old has passed away, the new has come.
2 Corinthians 5:17*

Paul teaches us that our spirits were made completely new at our salvation. However you may feel at times, spiritually you're seated with Christ in heavenly places, in a place of peace and rest.

For the sake of illustration, imagine a nation's capital city in the 1800's, when no cars, email, or even telephones existed, and suppose there were a change of government. The only way for that to get out to the surrounding area would be people on horses riding out to bring the news. Now the surrounding area would know pretty fast, but the far-flung states? And what about the little farmsteads and villages deep inside those states? It would be a good while before they heard the news, and were influenced by the changes in law that came with the new government.

The capital city represents your spirit. At salvation, we had a change of government, with a totally new way of thinking, speaking and doing life. For most of us, it takes the rest of our lives for that change of government to filter out to influence the rest of our souls. But we are already a new creation. This goes a long way to explain the apparent contradictions we see in scripture: we're saved by faith not works (Eph 2:8-9), but are called to work out our salvation (Eph 2:12); we are filled with His fullness (Col 2:10), but we will be filled as we come to know His love (Eph 3:19).

The implication of this is that we are now, at our core, made new. We are completely changed, we are the righteousness of Christ Jesus. Our identity is transformed. It is just a matter of teaching our souls that the government has changed. Inner healing goes a good way to do this, but we also need to agree with who God says we are and refuse behaviour, thoughts and belief systems that would be consistent with who we used to be.

Looking into Life

What has God said to you about who you are over your walk with Him, or through your ministry session?

_____
_____
_____
_____
_____
_____

Spend a few minutes with Him and ask Him what else He wants to tell you about you. Write down what He says here:

_____
_____
_____
_____
_____
_____

Are there any bits of the old you that have been trying to convince you they're still around or important? Are there any that you can shake off now, as you recognise they are no longer a part of who you are?

_____

_____

_____

_____

_____

_____

Take the truths that God's given you and turn them into declarations that you can make every morning. If it helps, put them up in prominent places by the mirror or on your cupboards, so that you're reminding yourself of them regularly.

Day 9: Who I Am

For as we have many members in one body, but all the members do not have the same function, so we, being many, are one body in Christ, and individually members of one another. Having then, gifts differing according to the grace that is given to us, let us use them.
Romans 12:4-6

You are unique. No one else has the same DNA, fingerprints, life experience or mix of giftings and skills as you. God's plan for us is glory: we were given it (John 17:22); born to reflect it and grow in it (2 Cor 3:18); and of course, each one of us reflects God's glory through the unique mosaic of our own make-up. That means that there are over seven billion aspects of God's glory currently being represented on the earth! No wonder the angels never run out of things to worship God for.

It is my belief that the only thing that holds us back is 'our revelation of God's revelation of us'- or our understanding of God's view of us. Once we know who we are, that is, we know ourselves as God sees us, then everything else can fall into place.

It is all too easy to define ourselves by what we do. For example, "I am a pastor, administrator, bank clerk." That's all great, but those labels are all about doing, rather than being. What we're looking for at this stage is what you'd look like if you never did another thing for God your whole life.

What does God say about the essence of who He made you to be?

I recall a British Bible teacher recounting an encounter he had with God, in which God showed the man himself as a construction site with rods and bricks and cement and mess. But God was describing the building as beautiful and architecturally stunning. The teacher couldn't match up the two scenes until God explained that He saw the man as the finished product, according to His blueprints as the architect. He was seeing him in his full potential, as who God made him to be.

Looking into Life

What has God said to you about your identity, and who you are?

_____
_____
_____
_____
_____

What has God said about who you are from previous prophetic words, or through His Word?

_____
_____
_____
_____
_____

How easy do you find it to agree with who He says you are?

_____
_____
_____

Ask God to show you what lies you're still believing in this area. What truth does He want to replace them with?

_____
_____
_____
_____

What would life look like in five years time if you believed the truth He's given you?

_____
_____
_____
_____

Reinforce this truth however it works for you: truth-reinforcing declarations on cards in your pocket or as reminders on your mobile.

Day 10: Sonship (Part I)

But when the fullness of the time had come, God sent forth His Son, born of a woman, born under the law, to redeem those who were under the law, that we might receive the adoption as sons. And because you are sons, God has sent forth the Spirit of His Son into your hearts, crying out, "Abba, Father!" Therefore you are no longer a slave but a son, and if a son, then an heir of God through Christ.
Galatians 4:4-7

In the story of the prodigal son in Luke 15, we read of a son who thought he was missing out and left home to find what he was missing, only to realise that no material thing could satisfy what he was looking for. Totally unprepared for what his father will do, he assumes he's blown it, but thinks he'll have a chance if he seeks to work his way back in. He tells his father, "I know I've probably blown it as your son, but please let me work for you as one of your hired men." Giving up the privileges of a son in his father's house, he figures at least he'll have a roof over his head and be around his Dad, albeit with shame hanging over him.

We read that story and think of it as purely evangelistic: a picture of the unbeliever receiving grace and mercy from God and being taken into his family. But it's also a picture of us as believers. Many of us may live on our Father's property, but we've never actually come home. Seemingly content with the servant's quarters, we attempt to get back into our Father's good graces by working for God, totally misunderstanding or forgetting that we're sons and daughters and our place is not with the servants but in the house, with access to the fridge and our Dad's cash, with no trace of shame in sight. We end up serving our Dad's vision whether we're sons or servants, but are invited to as sons, serving because we want to and we care about the family name and business. It's living from a place of inheritance. What we freely receive that someone else worked for- rather than from what we worked for.

Looking into Life

Where would you put yourself at the moment? Are you in the servants' quarters or in the Father's house?

_____
_____
_____

What is stopping you from embracing your position as a son or daughter?

- ☐ Performance
- ☐ Shame
- ☐ Fear of rejection
- ☐ Never realised it was available
- ☐ Fear of restriction or control
- ☐ Other_____

What does God want to tell you about this?

_____
_____
_____
_____

Is there anything else you need to forgive your own Dad for?

_____
_____

Ask God what life would look like for you if you gained a greater revelation of his Fatherhood.

_____
_____
_____
_____
_____

What evidence of your adoption into God's family can you see from the past week?

_____
_____
_____
_____

Declarations

God has chosen me to be his son or daughter.
Nothing I do can change my position as His child.
My Father delights in me, He dances over me
and is proud of me as His son or daughter.

Day 11: Sonship (Part II)

So he got up and came to his father. But while he was still a long way off, his father saw him and felt compassion for him, and ran and embraced him and kissed him.
Luke 15:20 (NASB)

Yesterday we saw that we're not slaves any longer, but stakeholders in the family business, which is the spreading abroad of God's kingdom on earth as it is in heaven. So what is the inheritance we received when we became sons?

Let's look back at Luke 15. The father gave his son a few things.

1. **Sandals.** In Jesus' day sons, not slaves, wore shoes. By giving his son sandals the father in the story was reinforcing that his son was still his son.

2. **A Cloak.** These are actually the best robes, reserved for honoured guests. With one act the son's shame was dealt with and he was put into a place of honour. The villagers no longer had a right to attack the son for his actions, instead they were invited to come and celebrate his return at a family party held in his honour.

3. **A Ring.** The ring given by a father to a son in that culture represented authority; with it a son would transact business in the name of the father and people had to treat him as they would have done his father.

What does this mean for us? It means we're not just sons, but we can stand tall. Our sins have been covered over, our shame washed away and our dignity restored. The enemy no longer has a right to accuse or shame us for past mistakes. Whenever he feeds us lies about our past, we can point to the cloak, the blood of Jesus, and silence him. We get to boldly approach the throne. Thirdly, we have authority. Our Father trusts us to do business in His name here on earth.

The journey into a place of honest and open sonship can last a lifetime, as we discover more and more about our incredible Father. Sometimes, though, it's us that holds this process up. If we've had a Dad who's let us down or hurt us we can subtly abort our place of sonship, and remove the place that a father stands in our hearts. Some would call it an inner vow, a decision like 'I've trusted a father once and he let me down so from now on I'll be the one who protects me' or 'I don't need authority over me or anyone to tell me what to do.' Most of the time this isn't a conscious decision, we just find it hard to find the place of a son or daughter, or don't get on well with authority figures in our lives. In these instances we will need to renounce any such vow we have made and deliberately both give ourselves permission to resume that place of sonship and rebuild the place for a father in our hearts.

Looking into Life

Are there any areas of your life where you're hanging on to shame? Take a few moments to ask God to reveal any area where it's still clinging on and give it to Him. What does He have for you in exchange? (Isa 61:7)

_____
_____
_____
_____

Where has God given you particular authority? If you're not sure take a few moments to ask Him.

_____
_____
_____

Are there any areas that He's given you authority in that you're hiding from, or have yet to start to walk out in? What lies do you believe that are keeping you from embracing them?

_____
_____
_____
_____ WALKING FREE _____

What more does God want to say to you about these areas?

_____
_____
_____
_____
_____

Could you have made an inner vow, or aborted your place of sonship? If so, renounce that vow now, give yourself permission to be a son or daughter again, and re-open that place in your heart for fathers to come and take their place in your life. What does Father God want to say to you about this? How does life look different from this new place?

_____
_____
_____
_____
_____
_____
_____
_____
_____

Day 12: The Power of Gratitude

Rejoice always, pray without ceasing, in everything give thanks; for this is the will of God in Christ Jesus for you.
1 Thessalonians 5:16-18

Rick Warren said it well: You were made for worship. You were made for worship like a fish was made for water. Fish look rather pathetic when on the ground, out of water, and actually, we look kinda sad and pathetic too, when we aren't breathing worship, specifically in the realm of thanksgiving. Things seem bigger and overwhelm us more when our heart's not exalting God and remembering how big He is. We get cynical and grow harder to the good in the world around us (which is evidence of God) when we don't take the time to acknowledge God in the midst of life's busyness.

The scientific world also recognises the power of thankfulness. In secular studies, an attitude of gratitude has been found to 'increase happiness by up to twenty-five percent, reduce stress and depression', and cause people to 'be more creative, bounce back faster from adversity, have a stronger immune system and have stronger social relationships' than those who don't practice gratitude.

No wonder provision was made for gratitude from the time offerings were first instituted (Exod 35:29). The Psalms sing out of a thankful heart, and we're told the entrance to God's presence is praise and thanksgiving (Psa 100:4); Jesus rewards gratitude (Luke 17:15-19); and Paul exhorts people to be thankful on many occasions (see 1Thess 5:18).

Do not underestimate the power of a thankful heart.

Looking into Life

What are you thankful for today?

_____
_____
_____
_____
_____
_____

How would you rate your current levels of thankfulness?
(1 = Not at all thankful, 10 = ecstatically thankful!)

1   2   3   4   5   6   7   8   9   10

Are there any areas in your life that could do with being infected by gratitude?

_____
_____
_____
_____

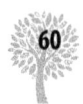

Try starting each day this week with 5 minutes of thankfulness, reminding yourself through the day to look for evidence of God's goodness.

I managed 5 minutes of thankfulness today! (Tick off as you go)

- ☐ Day 13
- ☐ Day 14
- ☐ Day 15
- ☐ Day 16
- ☐ Day 17
- ☐ Day 18
- ☐ Day 19

At the end of the week, on day 19, come back here and journal how it's affected you. Are you finding it easier to find things to be thankful for?

Day 13: The Normal Christian Life

And we know that all things work together for good to those who love God, to those who are the called according to [His] purpose.
Romans 8:28

Seasons. The normal Christian life is all about seasons. Not that summer all year wouldn't be delightful, it's just that it wouldn't really work too well because necessary things happen in spring, autumn and winter that just can't happen in summer time. If we're forewarned that life will have seasons it makes it much easier to traverse them well.

Remember those seasons when God feels close all the time? We're able to enter His presence in quiet times and worship times easily and the heavens seem open to our requests? You may be in one right now; if so, I'm celebrating with you! They're wonderful times. How about the seasons when He seems distant, we can't seem to feel His presence at all when people around us are having incredible experiences and the heavens seem like brass. If you're in one of those right now, hang in there, God is doing far more in you than you know.

If we don't realise that both seasons are part of the normal Christian life, we'll get into 'winters' and start asking questions like "What have I done wrong? Is there something I haven't repented of? Have I offended God?".

Once we're aware of the ebb and flow of normal life we can see that it is in these winter seasons that roots are going deeper and we are learning and developing truths and character traits that could never have been established in the summer times. In winter times we just need to spend more time huddling around the fire of His presence. The key in every season is to find out what it is that we would not have had the chance to learn if these life circumstances weren't happening, and then make sure we're partnering with Him to learn it fast! I love what Paul Manwaring of Bethel Church says: God makes such a good job of turning a situation around that it might even *look like* He sent it! Of course, we know that as a good Dad He never sends bad stuff to His kids.

Looking into Life

What season are you in at the moment? Is it a summer season or a winter one? A season of rest or a season of battle?

_____
_____
_____
_____
_____
_____

Ask Father God if there is anything you need to do to come into the present and embrace the season you're in. For example, taking off the war clothes and allowing yourself to rest, or stop striving to get back into summer and settle for winter for the time being?

_____
_____
_____
_____
_____
_____
_____

What do you feel God is teaching you through this season? If you're not sure ask Him!

_____
_____
_____
_____
_____

How can you partner with Him to do this season well?

_____
_____
_____
_____
_____

How will you know when this season is over?

_____
_____
_____
_____
_____

Day 14: Love

For this reason I bow my knees to the Father…that you, being rooted and grounded in love, may be able to comprehend with all the saints what is the width and length and depth and height- to know the love of Christ which passes all knowledge, that you may be filled with all the fullness of God.
Ephesians 3:14-19

It all comes down to love. Amazing, all-encompassing, fierce, pure, jealous, tender, patient, passionate, honouring, confident, sensitive, other-preferring, radiant, exuberant, understanding, enduring, long-suffering, fully accepting, penetrating, furious love. When Paul talks in One Corinthians thirteen about clanging cymbals and a life sacrificed for nothing, he's trying to get across just how vital love is to everything. It doesn't matter what were doing or how much we're doing it, if love isn't our motivation and it isn't Jesus' love that people see when they see us we've got more revelation to come. Thankfully the cry for a deeper experiential knowledge of love is one that God delights to answer, because as John tells us, we're actually asking for a deeper revelation of Him.

I have met a few people whose eyes shine with love, and I have asked them what made the difference, where love came from for them. Their answer has consistently been, "I had to learn to love myself first." Jesus did say, "love your neighbour as yourself" after all.

66

I'm so with you here: I'm learning more and more everyday what it looks like to live loved, and discovering the depths and the heights and the width of what perfect Love looks like. It is a journey with such an incredible reward—as if love itself were not enough! Being "filled with the fullness of God" awaits the one who throws himself open to the radical love of our extraordinary God and Father. Because no matter what you do, everything we are is based on the fact that we were fundamentally made not for what we can do, but to be objects of astonishing love.

Looking into Life

What things do you love? _____

_____

_____

What outcomes, or end results, do you love? _____

_____

_____

What do you love to do? _____

_____

_____

What can you celebrate about yourself as you look through what you love? To what extent do you find these things you love in yourself and in your life?

_____

_____

_____

What else do you see in yourself that you love?

_____

_____

What does God love about you? Why does He enjoy being around you so much?

_____
_____
_____

What is your number one barrier to a greater revelation of love? Ask God about it.

_____
_____
_____

What truth does God want to give you to bring that barrier down?

_____
_____
_____
_____

Spend some time soaking (putting on some quiet worship/soaking music and resting), focused on God and not trying to do anything, with no agenda other than to absorb God's love like a sponge.

Review of the Week

What are you thankful for this week?

_____
_____
_____
_____
_____

What spoke to you this week through your reading or God time?

_____
_____
_____
_____
_____

What have you learned about God through your reading or God time?

_____
_____
_____
_____

70

How will what you've learned this week affect day to day life from now on?

_____
_____
_____
_____
_____

Are there any loose ends you need to tie up from the past week? Anyone to forgive? Any steps forward to celebrate?

_____
_____
_____
_____
_____

Is there anything you want to run past God for the coming week? What did he tell you about it?

_____
_____
_____
_____

Day 15: Community

They devoted themselves to the apostles' teaching and to fellowship, to the breaking of bread and to prayer.
Acts 2:42

We were designed to live within the context of community. Community to live with, discover God's glory in, relate to, be supported by, engage with, love and be loved by. For one thing, community helps to meet our valid needs for comfort, encouragement and affirmation, so that in the times when we don't seem to be able to access God, we do not need to turn to unhealthy ways of getting those needs met.

Another important reason, though, is that community—being around and sharing with those around us, knowing others and being known by them—keeps us safe. Those isolated are easily picked off, and independence can lead to error all too fast. It is vital that we are in relationship with people who can speak into our lives and keep us accountable, let us know when we're off kilter and help us in the journey.

The problem with hurt people is that they hurt people, which makes community much harder. Broken people are often misunderstood, and often our own issues actually repel the very people we need, or we become over-dependent on others to meet the needs that we should be going to God to get met.

These are all reasons, though, why it is so important that we work to do community well. We need to step out of our comfort zones, reach out to others despite what we're feeling, and open up, within the context of safe relationship, to allow others in.

It is easy to get offended, but quite often offence, which rushes to blame others for their faults, is actually a red flag that there is something wrong with us. Living lifestyles of forgiveness and actively working on building trust with those around us are vital elements in building 'families' with low levels of anxiety (as Danny Silk would put it- see Appendix D). Relationships where we are free to be ourselves, and safe enough to allow others to see us for who we really are, are built over years of pursuing connection through peacetime and conflict, ups and downs.

Looking into Life

Who makes up your community?

_____
_____
_____
_____

On a more intimate level: who do you have that really knows you? Who around you speaks into your life?

_____
_____
_____
_____

If you don't have anyone, can you think of anyone that might be able to do this? If you're unsure ask God who He wants you to connect with, and how to go about that.

_____
_____
_____
_____

What can you do to reach a hand out to your community this week? It might be an individual who needs someone to talk to, a catch up with friends, or joining a group you have an interest in but have never been to before.

_____
_____
_____
_____

Is there any area of offence in your life at the moment that you need to talk to God about? What did He say/ what action do you need to take?

_____
_____
_____
_____

What do you think is your biggest boundary to doing community better? What is God saying to you about that?

_____
_____
_____
_____

Day 16: Looking After You

*I praise you because I am fearfully and wonderfully made,
Your works are wonderful. I know that full well...
Psalm 139:14*

Is it ok if I put my Doctor's hat on for a second? I've been so good and not told any nasty stories, or made you feel bad for that cake you ate yesterday. I'll put the hat away again really, really soon.

You are an incredible person. Seriously. I spent five years and a whole lot more hours scratching the surface of how incredible you are. You are a masterpiece of engineering and design, a breathtakingly beautiful work of architecture. You are a stunningly complex mix of God-design in genetics, experience, education and idiosyncrasy that work together to form *you*, the way you think and behave and react; the way you love and learn and relate. If you owned something as precious and intricate as *you*, you would look after it really well. Probably give it a tender polish every Saturday and buy the best oil you can from the workshop, spend that bit of extra money on Premium Unleaded, and choose your parking spaces very, very carefully.

Well, you know what I'm getting at. Very few of us look after our bodies as well as some guys treat the pride and joy that is their car. Unlike your car, though, you can't get spare parts so quickly and easily for you.

This is a friendly word from a doctor who's seen the evidence: please look after yourself. That looks like exercise, even if it's just walking a few times a week. It looks like putting decent fuel into your machine, not necessarily expensive or gourmet cuisine, just down-to-earth good-for-you high-nutritional-value food. It looks like drinking more water than anything else. It looks like getting decent amounts of sleep, and it looks like making time to enjoy other people, enjoy doing what you love, and make sure you're having fun. God made you for longevity and His plan for us is to walk in divine health, but as in most things with God it's all about partnership. Doing what we can to keep ourselves well spiritually, emotionally, mentally and physically puts us in the best possible position because we're running the machine (for want of a better word) as the creator's instruction manual suggests.

Looking into Life

How well do you look after yourself? If not well, why is that? Busyness is not an excuse for not looking after something precious- is there a lie you believe about yourself?

_____
_____
_____
_____

What is God telling you about any lie you're believing?

_____
_____
_____
_____

What one thing can you change this week to look after yourself better?

- ☐ *Make time for fun*
- ☐ *Get some early nights*
- ☐ *Drink more water*
- ☐ *Get out for some walks*
- ☐ *Convert to healthy snacks*
- ☐ *Meet up with friends*
- ☐ *Put away the soft drink!!!*
- ☐ *Eat breakfast*

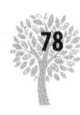

Do you have any physical illness? Spend some time asking God about it. Is there anything He wants to tell you?

_____
_____
_____
_____

Have you taken sensible precautions to ensure that you stay in good shape? Do you have a niggling problem that you need to see your doctor or a physiotherapist for? Have you been ignoring that skin lesion or bad back? Time to get it sorted! What will you do this week?

_____
_____
_____
_____

Take some time to schedule your next week or month. Plan in times to socialise and times to have fun, whatever that looks like to you.

Day 17: Embracing Process

For the vision is yet for the appointed time; It hastens towards the goal and it will not fail. Though it tarries, wait for it; It will certainly come, it will not delay.
Habakkuk 2:3 (NASB)

Process.

The very word makes many of us cringe. In our post-modern culture we are all about fast food, crash diets and instant downloads. The problem being that God doesn't seem to be in any sort of rush. Like a master craftsman, He takes whatever He finds in us and lovingly, painstakingly crafts us into something stunningly beautiful.

Most of our heroes in Scripture have been through this. Think of David. He was told he would be king, saw early success and then was on the run for fifteen years prior to finally taking his position on the throne. Or what about Joseph? A good life, good dreams, then it all takes a turn he hadn't expected and it's another thirteen years in slavery and imprisonment until his dreams finally come to pass. Or Paul? An incredible experience with God and then years missing in Arabia before he reappears to become the powerful man we know him as. Process. It's going to happen so we may as well embrace it.

Destination disease is commonplace among Christians. We see someone or something we want to be and expect to be there overnight. I remember going through this cycle over and over again in my teens. I'd get stirred by something, become desperately hungry for God, fast, pray and worship for hours for days, see nothing happen, get offended at God, cease to hear Him well, eventually realise I was offended, repent, and then have a short time of semi-normality before the whole thing repeated itself again. The whole cycle was exhausting, to say the least!

When we can rest in the knowledge that God has it covered and wants us to succeed more than we do, we can learn to take one day at a time. Then we will find it easier to find God quickly in every season and keep our focus on Him, taking us very quickly to where our hearts want to go. It's all about rest.

Looking into Life

Offence at God and others, impatience, jealousy and hopelessness are telltale signs of destination disease. Do any of these affect you? Spend some time with God dealing with them. What does He want you to know?

_____
_____
_____
_____
_____
_____

What is God saying to you about where you're at right now? What does He want to tell you about His promises over your life?

_____
_____
_____
_____
_____
_____
_____
_____

Are there any desires or promises that have been taking longer than you think, that you need to hand over to God?

_____
_____
_____
_____

As you look over your life over the last ten years what changes do you see in yourself? How have you changed for the better in the process of life over the last decade?

_____
_____
_____
_____

Spend some time thanking God for the changes you see.

Declarations
My times are in God's hands. He is leading me and guiding me in the way I should go.

I am moving from glory to glory as God crafts me to unlock who I am.

Day 18: Keeping The Enemy Foothold-Free

For if indeed I have forgiven anything, I have forgiven that one for your sakes in the presence of Christ, lest Satan should take advantage of us; for we are not ignorant of his devices.
2 Corinthians 2:10-11

In the 1940's, CS Lewis wrote an insightful, satirical book called *The ScrewTape Letters*. In it, the Demon Uncle is mentoring his nephew Wormwood in ways of interacting with his 'Patient' (a Christian) to try and ensure his damnation. It provides quite an insight into how the enemy works and what our lives as believers look like from his perspective. It is well worth the read, but for now we will take our own foray into the world of 'the enemy's devices'!

There are three main means of giving the enemy a foothold in our lives:

1. **Deliberate sin.** One of the most effective ways of ensuring that the enemy has a door into your world is to invite sin into your life. Now most of us wouldn't deliberately sin, but Hebrews four actually defines disobedience as refusing to listen to God, which reaches a whole lot wider, as it becomes not just what we are doing, but what God has told us to do and we shy away from.

2. **Agreement.** We've already dealt with this. Agreeing with the enemy's lies actually works as faith in him rather than faith in God, and gives the enemy authority that he previously did not have access to.

3. **Unforgiveness.** Withholding forgiveness from someone is another sure way of giving the enemy access and preventing us from functioning in a healthy way in that area. Many of us think that by not forgiving someone we hold them captive, not realising that it is actually us that's held captive by them. Whilst it may feel like forgiving someone is letting them off, it actually releases us to function as God intended. Some people even get physical healing when they forgive. It's just not worth holding on to things from the past. We have to walk in a lifestyle of forgiveness.

Looking into Life

Which of these three no-go-zones have you found the biggest problem with?

☐ Sin ☐ Agreement ☐ Unforgiveness

Ask God what He wants to say to you about any area where you're still struggling- write down what He said here:

_____
_____
_____
_____
_____

What action steps can you take to ensure you don't give the enemy a foothold in each of these areas?

Deliberate sin:_____
_____
_____
_____
_____

Wrong agreement: _____
_____
_____
_____
_____

Unforgiveness: _____
_____
_____
_____
_____

Declarations

I am a child of God, by God's grace I have everything I need to walk in righteousness.

*I live by faith and stand on God's truth.
I laugh at the lies of the enemy.*

*I walk in a lifestyle of forgiveness.
It's easy for me to forgive others.*

Day 19: When Trouble Comes

David was greatly distressed because the people spoke of stoning him, for all the people were embittered…But David strengthened himself in the Lord his God.
1 Samuel 30:6

If you've never had a hard season in your life it's ok, you can skip this page.

Oh, still reading? So it's not true that I'm the only one that goes through difficult times? But that's not what the enemy's told me. He's told me that everyone else is fine and I'm totally alone and no-one could possibly understand what I'm going through… Recognise the tactic?

It is a sad fact of life that, in this fallen world, we have trouble. I'm not being negative or making wrong confessions; these are Jesus' words, not mine! The second part of what He says is pretty crucial though, because if we ever stop at 'I'm in trouble' it can only lead to a bad day. Let's have a look at His words in John sixteen: "These things I have spoken to you, so that in me you may have peace." He's saying, "listen up guys- I'm about to give you quite a key here! 'In the world you have tribulation (see!), but take courage; I have overcome the world."

Wow! Most of us are rather good at identifying trouble, but what David found out, that we can rely on too, is that even in our darkest nights God has not changed, there has been no abdication in heaven, not one of His words to us have fallen, not one of our giftings has been revoked, His love never went anywhere. In short, circumstance has no power to get us off track, because like a GPS navigation system, when we take a wrong turn He just comes back with 'recalculating.' He's won, and as those called according to His purpose, we're in a very good place.

Of course, that doesn't mean that trouble doesn't feel like trouble! The trick seems to be being able to see things from God's perpective when hard times hit. Admittedly, sometimes when our world goes crazy we can't seem to find Him, and sometimes we can't hear what He's saying to us either. We do, however, always have the capacity to remember what He's said and who He is, and that, as David discovered, is our key.

Looking into Life

What are some things that God has told you that you can go back to when everything around you gets crazy? Maybe some of the things He told you about who you are, or the promises He's given you, or the memory of times when He has shown Himself to be a protector, provider or as the Healer.

_____
_____
_____
_____
_____
_____
_____
_____
_____
_____
_____
_____
_____
_____
_____

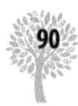

Start to accrue your pick-me-up collection!

- If you haven't already done so start a journal where you record what God's doing for you so that in times of trouble you can look back and strengthen yourself.

- Put some index cards together that you can carry with you so that you can remind yourself of who God says you are when things get tough. Write on them prophetic words you've received, God-encounters where He's affirmed or encouraged you, and key life verses.

- Start a thanks page. Add the little and big things that you're thankful for each day so that you end up with a thousand things to thank God for over time.

It's day 19! That means it's time to go back to day 12 and finish off the section on thankfulness.
You can use this space as a start-up thanks page until you get your own :-)

Day 20: Looking After Your Spirit

Watch your life and doctrine closely. Persevere in them, because if you do, you will save both yourself and your hearers.
1 Timothy 4:16

Well, we've tackled staying in physical health, but what about spiritual health? For a start, hopefully you've worked out by now that everything we do originates in love. The reason we look after our physical bodies is because we love ourselves and are deciding to steward what God has given us well, not because there's a set of rules to keep.

The same applies to our spirit. We actually do have to look after them for them to flourish. Both our spirit and our body require nourishment, nurture and exercise to become strong. Without time communing with God and constantly being filled with the Holy Spirit our spirit dries up; the power and awareness of God's presence that we're designed to carry start to fade. Without the food of God's word and solid teaching we become weak and easily swayed by any wind of doctrine—our strength and discernment fail. Paul describes it as being babies on milk when we should be on solid food.

We are not required to do anything, Jesus completely fulfilled the Law at the cross, meaning no further fulfilment is required from us.

However, as lovers of Jesus we will naturally want to protect His heart, so we'll deliberately put restrictions on ourselves to do that, just as one in love deliberately puts restrictions on himself to honour his partner. As Paul says, all things are permissible, but not all are wise.

There is no requirement, but the disciplines of daily prayer, worship and Bible reading actually build strength in our spirits, much in the same way as a regular commitment to the gym builds strength in our muscles.

Looking into Life

What does your God time look like?

Time. *Are you able to set aside time with God free of distractions? If no- what can you do to change this?*

_____
_____
_____
_____
_____

Prayer. *How do you come to God as you start? Do you come with requests, or turn your affections on Him and hear what He has to say first? Prayer is a two way process- to what extent does this apply to you?*

_____
_____
_____
_____
_____
_____
_____

Worship. *What form does your worship take? Are you able to make noise and truly express your heart to God? Try changing what you do every so often so that it stays fresh.*

_____

_____

_____

Bible study . *Do you study the Bible for yourself or do you depend on teaching books written by others? Getting our own revelation is so important. Are you following a Bible reading plan? If no, what are you doing to ensure that you cover the Bible in a balanced way (rather than sticking to your favourite books)? What can you do to bring new life to your Bible reading?*

_____

_____

_____

Is there anything else God wants to say to you about your times with Him?

_____

_____

_____

_____

Day 21: Onward Development

Congratulations! You made it through three weeks! By now your way of thinking has shifted and some of the things that you used to struggle with are fading into the distance. You're starting to implement change in many areas of your life that will lead to life, peace and a future that is brighter and stronger. You're on your way to knowing who you are and to discovering God's love for you.

But it doesn't stop here. This is only the beginning of a great adventure!

As you've gone through this booklet, certain things will have spoken to you amongst the many points. Whilst it is probably unrealistic to think that you'll be able to change everything at once, I would encourage you to pursue those topics that caught your attention through the further reading or links in the Appendix, and through other resources you may know.

In the past, you may have been used to a world where you had little control or felt like you were powerless. Part of the reason for this booklet is to show you that you are in control of your own life. Ultimately, only you are in charge of you, only you have responsibility for how you feel, think or behave, and only you can make the decisions that will change your world. As you make some of those decisions and start to partner with God you will move into more frequent seasons of growth and expansion, because a good steward is always trusted with increase.

Remember too that you have access to God. It sounds like common sense but experience has shown that it's not so common! We forget who He is, how much He knows, how close He is and how capable He is all too quickly. Whether we live in the truth of it or not, He does have the answers to whatever situation we find ourselves in at any given time, and He does want to help us.

Most of the time you'll be able to sort out rising issues directly with God, but if you do need someone to help you remember that's ok too. Stay vulnerable, stay in love and enjoy the ride!

Looking into Life

What topics have caught you over the past three weeks? Which would you like to pursue further?

_____
_____
_____
_____

How will you do this?

_____
_____
_____
_____
_____

Who might be able to help you or keep you accountable over this time?

_____
_____
_____
_____

What does God want to tell you about life from here on out?

_____
_____
_____
_____
_____

What declarations will you continue to declare over the coming weeks? You can check out Appendix C if you need some help.

_____
_____
_____
_____
_____
_____
_____
_____

Come back and reread your journey through Walking Free every six months for as long as you need. Being able to see your growth from this point will refresh and refocus you for the next season.

Appendices

A: Resources for Insight and Development
B: Extra truth sheets
C: Declarations
D: Further Reading and Resources
References

Appendix A:
Resources for Insight and Development

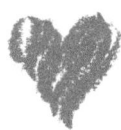

Heartlife Indicator
The product of 18 years of research by Stephen and Mara Klemich, the HeartLife Indicator is designed to help you see why you do what you do, or where your behaviour is coming from. It highlights those blind spots that we all have in character and attitude, utilising self-assessment and the assessment of those who know you to give honest feedback and ideas for lasting change for the good. Stephen and Mara have now given open access at no charge.

www.heartlifeindicator.com

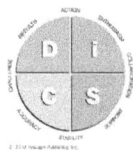

DISC Assessment
A secular tool that looks at your personality and how you interact with situations and people, seeking to shed light on why you do the things you do and how you can relate better to others.

DISC assessment available on the iBethel.org store

Dream Culture

A book, workbook and DVD series from Andy and Janine Mason, designed to unlock the hopes and dreams inside you, remove obstacles and get you moving towards your destiny.

Book and manual available from www.ibethel.org

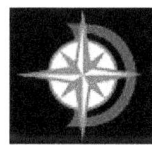

Destiny Finder

Again the result of a lot of research, destiny finder is an online profiling system created for Christian young adults (it works for anyone) that looks at your skills and giftings to give you insight into your make-up.

www.destinyfinder.com

Appendix B: Extra truth sheets

Truth Sheet

Write your truth from your ministry session here:

_____
_____
_____

Can you remember how God gave you this truth? Was it a sense or a picture, did you hear it or feel it?

_____
_____

What lie was it replacing?

_____
_____
_____

How has it been since you received this truth? Has the lie tried to get you again? How did you do standing on the truth?

_____
_____
_____

Spend a few minutes meditating on (asking God about) this truth. What else did He tell you about it?

_____
_____
_____
_____
_____

What would your life look like in a year if you believed this truth?

_____
_____
_____
_____
_____

What can you declare to reinforce this truth in your life?

_____
_____
_____
_____

Truth Sheet

Write your truth from your ministry session here:

_____
_____
_____

Can you remember how God gave you this truth? Was it a sense or a picture, did you hear it or feel it?

_____
_____

What lie was it replacing?

_____
_____
_____

How has it been since you received this truth? Has the lie tried to get you again? How did you do standing on the truth?

_____
_____
_____

Spend a few minutes meditating on (asking God about) this truth. What else did He tell you about it?

_____
_____
_____
_____
_____

What would your life look like in a year if you believed this truth?

_____
_____
_____
_____
_____

What can you declare to reinforce this truth in your life?

_____
_____
_____
_____

Truth Sheet

Write your truth from your ministry session here:

_____
_____
_____

Can you remember how God gave you this truth? Was it a sense or a picture, did you hear it or feel it?

_____
_____

What lie was it replacing?

_____
_____
_____

How has it been since you received this truth? Has the lie tried to get you again? How did you do standing on the truth?

_____
_____
_____

Spend a few minutes meditating on (asking God about) this truth. What else did He tell you about it?

_____
_____
_____
_____
_____

What would your life look like in a year if you believed this truth?

_____
_____
_____
_____
_____

What can you declare to reinforce this truth in your life?

_____
_____
_____
_____

Appendix C: Declarations

1. My prayers are powerful and effective (2 Cor 5:21; James 5:16b).

2. God richly supplies all my financial needs (Phil 4:19).

3. I am dead to sin and alive to obeying God (Romans 6:11).

4. I walk in ever-increasing health (Isaiah 53:3-5).

5. I live under a supernatural protection (Ps 91).

6. I prosper in all my relationships (Luke 2:52)

7. I consistently bring God encounters to other people (Mark 16:17,18)

8. Through Jesus I am 100% loved and worthy to receive all of God's blessings (Gal 3:1-5).

9. Each of my family members is wonderfully blessed and radically loves Jesus (Acts 16:30.31)

10. I uproariously laugh when I hear a lie from the devil (Psalms 2:2-4).

For further example declarations see ibethel.org.

Write your own declarations here:

_____
_____
_____
_____
_____
_____
_____
_____
_____
_____
_____
_____
_____
_____
_____
_____
_____
_____
_____

Appendix D: Further Reading and Resources

^ *Available at the iBethel store*

Day 1
- *Hearing God's Voice (Audio)- Bill Johnson* ^
- *You May All Prophesy (Book)- Steve Thompson*^
- *Can You Imagine? Why imagination is crucial to the Christian Life. (Article)*
- *Brandon J O'Brien. Christianity Today. or www.christianitytoday.com/biblestudies/articles/theology/canyouimagine.html?start=4*

Day 2
- *Relentless Mind Renewal (Audio)- Steve Backlund*^

Days 3 and 4
- *Fear is Not Your Friend (Audio)- Kris Vallotton*^
- *The Happy Intercessor (Book)- Beni Johnson*^
- *The Three Battlegrounds (Book)- Francis Frangipane*
- *Warring Wisely (Audio)- Kate Jutsum*

Day 5
- *Battlefield of the Mind (Book)- Joyce Meyer*

- *Let's Just Laugh At That (Book)- Steve Backlund^*

Day 6
- *Declarations: Unlocking Your Future (Book) - Steve Backlund^*
- *Declarations Make a Difference. (Article) Kevin Dedmon. www.ibethel.org/articles/2009/07/20/declarations-make-a-difference.*
- *Why We Make Declarations (Audio)- Steve Backlund^*
- *You're crazy if you don't talk to yourself (Book)- Steve Backlund^*

Day 7
- *Life's Journey from a Place of Rest (Audio)- Kate Jutsum*
- *Out of Striving, into Rest (Audio)- Seth Dahl^*

Day 8
- *The New Creation Miracle (Book) Phil Mason*
- *Towards a Powerful Inner Life (Book) Graham Cooke*

Day 9
- *Discovering and Impacting Your World (Audio)- Paul Manwaring^*
- *The Art of Being You (Book) Bob Kilpatrick and Joel Kilpatrick^*

Days 10-11
- *Daddy, You love me (Book) - Brent Lokker*
- *Father of Lights (Movie)- Darren Wilson^*
- *Glorious Sons and Daughters (Audio) - Paul Manwaring^*

- *When Law Met Love (Audio)- Kate Jutsum*

Day 12
- *Thanks!: How Practicing Gratitude Can Make You Happier (Book)- Robert Emmons*
- *The Supernatural Power of Thanksgiving (Audio)- Chris Overstreet^*

Day 13
- *Hiddenness and Manifestation (Book)- Graham Cooke*
- *The Calling Journey (Workbook)- Tony Stolzfuz^*

Day 14
- *Furious Love (Movie)- Darren Wilson^*
- *Journey of Love and Grace (Audio)- Chris Overstreet^*

Day 15
- *Community (Audio)- Banning Liebscher^*
- *Keep Your Love On (Book)- Danny Silk^*
- *Living a Life Unoffendable (Audio)- Dawna DeSilva**

Day 16
- *Supernatural Rest (Audio)- Bill Johnson^*

Day 17
- *No Longer Infants (Audio)- Kate Jutsum*
- *Enjoying Where you are on the way to where you are going (Book)- Joyce Meyer*

Day 18
- *Tactics of the Enemy (Audio)- Dawna DeSilva*
- *The Screwtape Letters (Book)- CS Lewis*

Day 19
- *Strengthen Yourself in the Lord (Book)- Bill Johnson*
- *See, Hear, Remember (Audio)- Bill Johnson*

Day 20
- *Changing Your World (Audio)- Bill Johnson^*
- *Hosting the Presence (Book)- Bill Johnson^*
- *This Present Presence (Audio)- Paul Manwaring^*

Day 21
- *On the Road to Destiny (Audio)- Dawna DeSilva and Faith Blatchford*
- *See also Appendix A*

References

Day 1.
- John 10:27

Day 2.
- Amos 3:7, Isaiah 59:16
- Strongs G342
- Engaging Families in the Early Childhood Development Story. Pam Winter. Education Services Australia. 2010.
- Mohs, Richard C.. "How Human Memory Works" 08 May 2007. HowStuffWorks.com. <http://science.howstuffworks.com/life/inside-the-mind/human-brain/human-memory.htm> 05 August 2013.

Day 3.
- The Three Battlegrounds. 2006. Francis Frangipane. Arrow Publications,
- Proverbs 23:7, Eph 6:12-18, Ephesians 3:10, Matt 6:9-13

Day 4.
- Hebrews 11, 1 John 4:18, Joshua 2:11, Judges 7:3

Day 7.
- Skeletal Muscle Damage and Repair. Peter M. Tildus. Human Kinetics, 2008.

Day 9.
- Judson Cornwall, preaching in 1982. No known written source.

Days 10-11.
- Luke 15:11-32
- The Cross and the Prodigal: Luke 15 through Middle Eastern Eyes. Kenneth E. Bailey. Intervarsity Press, 2005,
- Hebrews 4:16

Day 12.
- The Purpose Driven Life. Rick Warren. Zondervan, 2002,
- Thanks!: How Practicing Gratitude Can Make You Happier (Book)- Robert Emmons

Day 14.
- Leviticus 19:18, quoted by Jesus and Paul through the NT

Day 18.
- Hebrews 4:1-7, Matthew 18:23-31

Day 20.
- For a fuller discussion on the subject of the Law ref. Resources

www.ingramcontent.com/pod-product-compliance
Lightning Source LLC
Chambersburg PA
CBHW061332040426
42444CB00011B/2879